The Stomach Care Handbook

Unlock the Secrets to a Healthy Digestive System

BY

JOSEPH EDWARDS JNR

TABLE OF CONTENT

CHAPTER ONE INTRODUCTION 5

CHAPTER TWO UNDERSTANDING THE DIGESTIVE SYSTEM11

CHAPTER THREE THE STOMACH SOLUTION PRINCIPLES 15

CHAPTER FOUR COMMON DIGESTIVE DISORDERS AND SOLUTIONS 25

CHAPTER FIVE STOMACH-FRIENDLY RECIPES AND MEAL PLANS 33

CHAPTER SIX STOMACH CARE FOR DIFFERENT LIFE STAGES AND CONDITIONS 54

CHAPTER SEVEN RECIPES FOR A HEALTHY DIGESTIVE SYSTEM 74

CHAPTER EIGHT SUPPLEMENTS AND DIGESTIVE HEALTH80

CHAPTER NINE CASE STUDIES AND SUCCESS STORIES 86

CHAPTER TEN CONCLUSION 89

CHAPTER ONE

INTRODUCTION

Welcome to the "Stomach Care Handbook," an extensive manual for understanding and sustaining your body's essential stomach-related organs. Your stomach assumes a critical role in handling the food varieties you eat, engrossing fundamental supplements, and keeping up with, generally speaking, wellbeing of the whole man.

In this handbook, we will investigate the complex operations of the stomach, uncover normal stomach-related issues, and develop functional systems for advancing stomach-related well-being. From the second you take your most memorable chomp of food, your stomach starts its multifaceted dance of absorption, separating complex sugars, proteins, and fats to remove the energy and supplements your body needs to flourish.

In any case, what happens when this cycle is disturbed? This handbook means to respond to that inquiry and proposition answers to guarantee your stomach keeps on working at its ideal. Whether you have encountered infrequent stomach-related distress or need to proactively care for your stomach, this handbook is intended to engage you with information and viable tips.

We will embark on a journey to discover the factors that contribute to optimal digestive health through holistic stomach care, lifestyle choices, and dietary choices. Go along with us as we dive into the mind-boggling universe of stomach care, where you will acquire important bits of knowledge, learn compelling procedures, and leave on a path towards sustaining your body from the inside.

Let the "Stomach Care Handbook" be your personal compendium toward stomach-related health.

Sound-Stomach-Related Framework: The human stomach-related framework is comprised of incredible intricacy and effectiveness; dealing with the breakdown and ingestion of fundamental supplements for supporting life is critical.

The stomach is one of the most important parts of the human body. It is a biochemical powerhouse that is in charge of fully assimilating the nutrients that are needed and are important for overall digestive health. Inside this book, "The Stomach Care Handbook" it opens the key to a solid Stomach-Related Framework.

We will set out on an excursion to disentangle the complexities of the stomach-related process, focusing on the stomach's importance and its effect on our wellbeing. This guide isn't simply a gathering of realities and speculations; it is a pragmatic guide intended to engage you with the information and devices to cultivate a hearty stomach-related framework in the event that the directions are followed with the help of medical care experts.

The Importance of Having a Grasp in Good Health: The excursion starts with an investigation of why stomach-related wellbeing is central to our general health. We dig into the interconnections of the stomach-related framework with different physical processes, underscoring how a solid stomach sets the foundation for ideal supplement ingestion, energy creation, and invulnerable framework support.

From the osmosis of essential supplements to the disposal of waste, each aspect of our wellbeing is complicatedly attached to the proficiency of our stomach-related framework.

Outline of the Stomach Care Guide: More than just a guide, the stomach care handbook takes a holistic approach to digestive health. The fundamental ideas that will be discussed in the subsequent chapters are outlined in this section. We present the meaning of sustenance and diet, the effect of way of life decisions, and the joining of all encompassing practices into a sound stomach-related framework.

The Stomach Arrangement is certainly not a one-size-fits-all cure, yet it is an adaptable plan that perceives individual contrasts and gives commonsense, significant bits of knowledge. As we set out on this investigation, remember that accomplishing a sound stomach-related framework isn't just about lessening side effects; it's about cultivating a way of life that advances and supports wellbeing.

Through figuring out the job of the stomach and carrying out the standards of the stomach arrangement, you're not only opening the key to stomach-related well-being; you're also developing an establishment for an energetic and versatile life. Go along with us on this illuminating excursion as we demystify the complexities of the stomach and uncover the keys to stomach-related imperativeness.

CHAPTER TWO

UNDERSTANDING THE DIGESTIVE SYSTEM

Life Structures of the Intestinal System: The intestinal system, otherwise called the gastrointestinal lot, is a mind-boggling framework answerable for separating food and engrossing supplements.

The mouth: It begins from the mouth and incorporates the throat, stomach, small digestive system, internal organ, rectum, and rear end. Mouth: The stomach-related process starts here, where food is bitten and blended in with spit to start the breakdown of mind-boggling sugars.

Esophagus: Through contractions known as peristalsis, this muscular tube carries food from the mouth to the stomach.

Stomach: The stomach is a solid organ that fills in as a brief stockpiling site for food. It secretes gastric juices, including acids and proteins, as an additional separate food.

Small Digestive Tract: The small digestive system is where the greater part of the assimilation and supplement ingestion happen. It consists of three sections: the duodenum, jejunum, and ileum.

Internal organ: Otherwise called the colon. The digestive organ ingests water and electrolytes from undigested food, shaping strong waste (dung).

Rectum and Rear- End: The rectum stores dung until it is prepared for disposal through the butt.

Job of the Stomach in Absorption: The stomach assumes an urgent part in the stomach-related process. Here are its primary capabilities:

Capacity: The stomach can grow to accommodate an enormous volume of food, permitting slow delivery into the small digestive tract for ideal processing.

Mechanical and Compound Assimilation: The stomach's strong constrictions stir and blend food in with gastric juices, separating it truly and synthetically.

Corrosive Creation: The stomach secretes hydrochloric corrosive, which helps kill microbes and separate proteins into more modest atoms.

Catalyst Emission: The stomach discharges compounds, for example, pepsin, which start the breakdown of proteins into peptides.

Normal stomach-related issues: Stomach-related issues can happen because of different elements.

The following are a couple of normal issues:

Indigestion: Otherwise called GERD, this happens when stomach corrosive streams once more into the throat, causing acid reflux and inconvenience.

Crabby Gut Condition (IBS): IBS is a constant gastrointestinal problem characterized by stomach torment, swelling, and changes in gut propensities.

Gastritis: Gastritis is the irritation of the stomach lining, frequently brought about by contamination, inordinate liquor utilization, or certain drugs. The run is a typical intestinal problem characterized by successive, free, and watery defecations.

Understanding the stomach-related framework lays the foundation for fathoming the mind-boggling processes that unfurl inside our bodies. From the underlying phases of rumination in the mouth to the retention of fundamental supplements in the small digestive tract, each portion of the gastrointestinal system assumes a significant role. The stomach, specifically, arises as a vital participant in coordinating processing and preparing for supplement digestion.

As we push ahead in "The Stomach Care Guide," the comprehension of the stomach-related framework will act as the bedrock for carrying out systems and way of life changes that cultivate a sound and tough stomach-related climate.

By unwinding the privileged insights of processing, we enable ourselves to make informed decisions that decisively influence our general prosperity.

CHAPTER THREE

THE STOMACH SOLUTION PRINCIPLES

Healthy Eating Habits: are behaviors and choices that help people feel and look their best through food. A few vital parts of good dieting propensities include:

Balanced Diet: Devouring various supplement-rich food sources from all significant nutritional categories, including natural products, vegetables, entire grains, lean proteins, and solid fats.

Portion Control: Being aware of piece sizes to forestall gorging and keep a sound weight.

Limiting Processed Foods: Limiting the admission of vigorously processed food sources that are ordinarily high in added sugars, undesirable fats, and sodium.

Hydration: remaining satisfactorily hydrated by drinking adequate amounts of water over the course of the day.

Mindful Eating: Focusing on yearning and totality signs, eating gradually, and relishing the kinds of food.

By embracing good dieting propensities, you can uphold ideal sustenance, keep a solid weight, and decrease the risk of ongoing illnesses.

Significance of Fiber: Fiber is a sort of carbohydrate found in plant-based food sources that can't be separated by the human stomach-related framework. It assumes an urgent role in keeping a solid stomach-related framework and offers a few advantages, for example:

Digestive Health: Dietary fiber adds mass to the stool, advancing normal solid discharges and preventing obstruction. It likewise assists with maintaining a good arrangement of stomach microscopic organisms.

Blood Sugar Management: Fiber slow down the assimilation and retention of sugar, prompting more steady glucose levels.

Weight Management: Food sources high in fiber will generally be seriously filling, which can assist with controlling cravings and advancing weight loss.

Heart Well-being: Particular sorts of fiber, like solvent fiber, can assist with bringing down cholesterol levels, in this way decreasing the risk of coronary illness.

Disease Prevention: Consuming enough fiber has been linked to a lower risk of a number of conditions, including diverticular disease, type 2 diabetes, and some types of cancer. To get enough fiber in your diet, it's best to eat a variety of fruits, vegetables, whole grains, legumes, and nuts.

Role of Probiotics: Probiotics are live microorganisms, frequently alluded to as "great microbes," that give medical advantages when consumed in satisfactory amounts. They can have a number of advantages, such as:

Digestive Health: Probiotics help reestablish and maintain a good overall arrangement of stomach microbes, which is fundamental for ideal processing and supplement ingestion. They can likewise support the administration of different circumstances, including:

Gastrointestinal Issues: Probiotics have been shown to mitigate the side effects of stomach-related illnesses like bad-tempered inside disorder (IBS), incendiary entrail infection (IBD), and the flu.

Immune System Support They can assist with fortifying the insusceptible framework and lessen the risk of respiratory contaminations, like the normal cold or influenza.

Emotional well-being: rising research recommends that probiotics might emphatically affect emotional wellness conditions like uneasiness and despondency.

Skin Health: Acne, eczema, and dermatitis can all be alleviated with probiotics.

Women's Health: Certain kinds of probiotics can help keep a solid vaginal microbiota and decrease the risk of urinary tract contamination and yeast diseases. To integrate probiotics into your eating routine, you can devour mature food varieties like yogurt, kefir, sauerkraut, and kimchi, or consider taking a probiotic supplement.

Stress Management: Stress on the board includes carrying out procedures and methods to adapt to and diminish the adverse consequences of weight on your psychological and actual prosperity. Some important points:

Deep breathing exercises: Profound breathing initiates the body's unwinding reaction, decreasing pressure and nervousness. You can attempt strategies like diaphragmatic breathing or 4-7-8 relaxing.

Engaging in enjoyable activities: Partaking in exercises you enjoy can assist with diverting your psyche from stressors and advance unwinding. Whether it's perusing a book, painting, or playing an instrument, find something that gives you pleasure and set aside a few minutes for it.

Mindfulness and meditation: These practices include concentrating on the current second, advancing, unwinding, and lessening pressure. You can attempt directed reflection applications or go to care classes for direction.

Adequate sleep: Getting sufficient quality rest is essential for managing feelings of anxiety. Hold back no longer than long stretches of rest each evening, and lay out a sleep-time routine to assist with loosening up your brain and body before rest.

Regular Physical Activity: Ordinary active work has various advantages for both physical and mental prosperity. You ought to know this:

Types of exercise: Perform a combination of cardiovascular exercises, such as swimming, walking, jogging, and weightlifting, and strength training exercises, such as bodyweight exercises, to build muscle and improve overall fitness. **Recommended duration:** Hold back nothing—150 minutes of moderate-force oxygen-consuming activity or 75 minutes of lively power work out, spread over time. It's likewise beneficial to consolidate strength-building practices no less than two times per week.

Benefits: Standard active work can lessen the risk of ongoing infections, support state of mind, further develop rest quality, increase energy levels, and generally improve prosperity.

Safety considerations: Focus on your wellbeing while working out. Begin with exercises that match your wellness level, warm up before exercises, and cool down subsequently. Before beginning a new exercise routine, consult a healthcare professional if you have any health concerns.

Adequate Hydration Legitimate hydration is fundamental for keeping up with different physical processes and, generally speaking, wellbeing. This is the very thing you ought to remember:

Water intake: Expect to drink around 8 cups (64 ounces) of water each day. Nonetheless, individual requirements might differ in light of variables, for example, environment, movement level, and, generally speaking, wellbeing. Pay attention to your body's thirst flags and change as needed.

Advantages of hydration: Remaining hydrated upholds legitimate processing, supplement retention, temperature guidelines, joint grease, and generally physical processes. It can also improve mood, energy, and cognitive function.

Tips for staying hydrated: Convey a refillable water bottle with you over the course of the day as a suggestion to routinely hydrate. Put forth objectives or use hydration following applications to screen your admission. In the event that you battle to hydrate, mix it with natural products or spices for a reviving character.

Signs of dehydration: Dry mouth, dark urine, fatigue, dizziness, or headaches, is crucial. Assuming that you experience these side effects, increment your liquid admission instantly. Keep in mind that sustaining a healthy, well-balanced lifestyle is a journey that requires persistence and patience.

It's critical to stand by listening to your body's requirements, focus on taking care of oneself, and roll out slow improvements that line up with your objectives. Assuming that you want further direction or have additional inquiries, go ahead and inquire!

Normal stomach-related diseases present special difficulties, yet understanding their causes and side effects is the most important step toward successful administration.

For heartburn and GERD, ways of life change, and drugs can mitigate side effects. Dietary adjustments, stress reduction, and, in some instances, medication are all components of IBS management. Crohn's disease and ulcerative colitis are examples of inflammatory bowel diseases that necessitate a multidisciplinary treatment plan that may include medication, dietary modifications, and even surgery.

Individualized care and an exhaustive comprehension of these issues engage people to explore their stomach-related wellbeing venture. Looking for proficient exhortation, taking on a fitted way to deal with way of life and diet, and remaining informed about accessible medicines are pivotal parts of overseeing normal stomach-related messes.

CHAPTER FOUR

COMMON DIGESTIVE DISORDERS AND SOLUTIONS

A. Heartburn and GERD:

Acid reflux occurs when stomach acid rises again into the esophagus, causing irritation and discomfort. Gastroesophageal reflux infection (GERD) alludes to ongoing indigestion. Normal causes include a powerless lower esophageal sphincter (the muscle that keeps the stomach corrosive from streaming back up), hiatal hernia (when the upper piece of the stomach pushes through the stomach), weight, pregnancy, and certain prescriptions. Heartburn, regurgitation, chest pain, difficulty swallowing, coughing, and a sour taste in the mouth are all possible signs.

Dietary and Way of Life Changes

To oversee indigestion and GERD, it's useful to make specific dietary and lifestyle changes. A few hints include: Avoiding trigger foods: Acid reflux can be triggered by a number of foods, including citrus fruits, tomatoes, fatty and fried foods, chocolate, mint, caffeine, and alcohol. Identifying and avoiding these trigger foods is beneficial.

Eating smaller, more frequent meals

Consuming more modest parts can assist with lessening tension on the stomach and limit heartburn side effects. Keeping a solid weight: Overabundance weight can come down on the stomach, adding to indigestion. Keeping a solid load through ordinary activity and a reasonable eating regimen can lessen side effects.

Elevating the head while sleeping

Raising the top of your bed or utilizing a wedge cushion can assist with keeping stomach corrosive from streaming once more into the throat while you rest.

Stopping smoking

Smoking debilitates the lower esophageal sphincter and can worsen indigestion side effects. Quitting smoking can help alleviate acid reflux and improve overall health.

B. Peevish Gut Condition (IBS):

Grasping IBS: A bad-tempered gut condition is a typical stomach-related jumble that influences the internal organs. The specific reason for IBS is obscure; however, factors like strange muscle constrictions in the digestive organs, over-sensitivity of the stomach, irritation, and changes in stomach microorganisms might contribute. The side effects of the IBS shift, however ordinarily, incorporate stomach torment, bulging, gas, the runs, and obstruction. Symptoms can be sparked or exacerbated by stress or certain foods.

Overseeing IBS through Diet and Way of Life: While there is no solution for IBS, dietary and lifestyle changes can assist with managing side effects, including:

Identifying trigger foods

Keeping a food journal can assist with distinguishing explicit food sources that trigger side effects. Normal triggers incorporate hot food varieties, greasy food sources, caffeine, and liquor.

Increasing fiber intake: Step by step, expanding fiber in your eating routine can assist with managing defecations and lessen stoppage or looseness of the bowels. Nonetheless, certain individuals with IBS are sensitive to particular kinds of fiber, so it's essential to investigate and find what turns out best for you. Dis solvable fiber, found in food varieties like oats, bananas, and root vegetables, is many times better endured.

Drinking a lot of water

Remaining hydrated is significant for keeping up with sound processing and preventing obstruction. to hydrate over the course of the day.

Managing stress

Stress is a known trigger for IBS side effects. Participating in pressure-lessening exercises like activity, reflection, profound breathing activities, or leisure activities can assist with managing side effects. If necessary, think about talking with a specialist or guide for extra help.

Regular physical activity

Taking part in ordinary activity can assist with directing solid discharges and decrease the side effects of IBS. Pick exercises that you appreciate, like strolling, yoga, or swimming.

Eating smaller, more frequent meals

Consuming a lot of food can put extra strain on the digestive system. Eating more modestly, even dinners over the course of the day, can help forestall the setting off of side effects.

Probiotics

Probiotics are gainful microscopic organisms that can assist with reestablishing the equilibrium of stomach verdure. They are accessible in supplement structure or can be found in specific food varieties like yogurt, sauerkraut, or kimchi. Examine with your PCP or an enlisted dietitian prior to beginning any new enhancements.

Avoiding triggers

Certain foods and drinks, such as spicy foods, carbonated beverages, foods high in fat, and those sweetened with artificial sweeteners, can make symptoms worse. Recognizing and staying away from your own triggers can be useful.

Looking for help

Living with IBS can be testing, but you're in good company. You might want to think about joining online communities or support groups where you can meet people who understand what you're going through.

Keep in mind that it means a lot to work with your medical services supplier or an enlisted dietitian to foster a customized plan for dealing with your IBS side effects. They can provide guidance and support based on your specific needs.

CHAPTER FIVE

STOMACH-FRIENDLY RECIPES AND MEAL PLANS

A collection of food options and dietary plans specifically designed to support digestive health and a comfortable stomach are referred to as stomach-friendly recipes and meal plans. These recipes and dinner plans are created with fixings and cooking strategies that are delicate on the stomach, making them reasonable for people who might encounter stomach-related issues or distress.

Here are a few qualities and standards frequently connected with stomach-accommodating recipes and dinner plans: Simple-to-Process Fixings: Emphasis on foods that are whole and minimally processed. Incorporation of effectively edible proteins, like lean meats, fish, and plant-based proteins. Joining of low-fat dairy or dairy choices.

Fiber-Rich Foods:

Integration of high-fiber ingredients like fruits, vegetables, whole grains, and legumes to support digestive regularity.

Anti-Inflammatory Components:

Use of ingredients with anti-inflammatory properties, such as ginger, turmeric, and certain herbs, to soothe the digestive system.

Balanced Nutrition:

A focus on a well-balanced mix of macro nutrients (carbohydrates, proteins, and fats) and micro-nutrients (vitamins and minerals) for overall health.

Hydration:

Encouragement to stay adequately hydrated to support the digestive process and prevent constipation.

Probiotics and Prebiotics:

Incorporation of foods rich in probiotics (live beneficial bacteria) and prebiotics (substances that promote the growth of beneficial bacteria) to support a healthy gut microbiome.

Mindful Cooking Methods

Inclination for cooking strategies that are delicate on the stomach, like baking, steaming, or sauteing, instead of broiling or weighty handling.

Adaptations of Traditional Dishes

Change of customary recipes to make them more stomach-accommodating without compromising flavor or social importance.

Meal Planning Strategies

Structured meal plans with a variety of flavors and nutrients for the day. Thought of part sizes and dividing dinners to forestall indulging and advance stomach-related solace.

Individualized Approaches.

Confirmation that various people might have extraordinary dietary necessities and responsive qualities, empowering a customized way to deal with stomach-accommodating eating. Recipes and meal plans that are easy on the stomach can be helpful for people who suffer from irritable bowel syndrome (IBS), acid reflux, or general digestive discomfort.

They want to give you options that are filling and good for your digestive system. Keep in mind that every person has different dietary requirements, and working with a nutritionist or other health care professional can give you specific advice based on your specific health concerns and goals.

Delicious and Nourishing Recipes for Supporting Digestive Health

Delicious and Nourishing Recipes for Supporting Digestive Health are dinners that are delectable as well as explicitly created to advance a solid stomach-related framework. These recipes regularly integrate fixings that are known for their stomach-related benefits, for example, those with mitigating properties, high fiber content, and supplements that help stomach wellbeing. Here are instances of such recipes:

Ginger and Turmeric Smoothie:

Ingredients:

Fresh ginger

Turmeric

Spinach

Banana

Greek yogurt

Almond milk

Benefits:

Ginger and turmeric have anti-inflammatory properties.

Yogurt provides probiotics for a healthy gut.

Quinoa Salad with Avocado and Chickpeas:

Ingredients:

Quinoa

Avocado

Chickpeas

Cherry tomatoes

Cucumber

Olive oil and lemon dressing

Benefits:

Quinoa is a whole grain with fiber.

Avocado provides healthy fats.

Chickpeas contribute protein and fiber.

Baked Chicken with Rosemary and Lemon:

Ingredients:

Chicken breast

Fresh rosemary

Lemon

Garlic

Olive oil

Benefits:

Baking preserves the nutritional content of the chicken.

Lemon adds a refreshing flavor and vitamin C.

Mango and Papaya Smoothie Bowl:

Ingredients:

Mango

Papaya

Greek yogurt

Chia seeds

Almond butter

Benefits:

Mango and papaya contain digestive enzymes.

Chia seeds provide omega-3 fatty acids.

Salmon and Quinoa Stuffed Bell Peppers:

Ingredients:

Salmon

Quinoa

Bell peppers

Spinach

Feta cheese

Benefits:

Salmon offers omega-3 fatty acids.

Quinoa is a good source of protein and fiber.

Lentil and Vegetable Soup:

Ingredients:

Lentils

Carrots

Celery

Spinach

Vegetable broth

Benefits:

Lentils are rich in fiber and protein.

Vegetables provide essential vitamins and minerals.

Yogurt Parfait with Berries and Almonds:

Ingredients:

Greek yogurt

Mixed berries (blueberries, strawberries)

Almonds

Honey

Benefits:

Greek yogurt offers probiotics.

Berries are rich in antioxidants.

Turkey and Quinoa Stuffed Acorn Squash:

Ingredients:

Ground turkey

Quinoa

Acorn squash

Onion

Garlic

Benefits:

Turkey is a lean protein source.

Quinoa adds fiber and nutrients.

Spinach and Mushroom Omelette:

Ingredients:

Eggs

Spinach

Mushrooms

Feta cheese

Benefits:

Spinach provides iron and fiber.

Eggs offer high-quality protein.

Chia Seed Pudding with Kiwi and Coconut:

Ingredients:

Chia seeds

Coconut milk

Kiwi

Shredded coconut

Benefits:

Chia seeds are rich in fiber and omega-3 fatty acids.

Coconut milk adds a creamy texture.

The goal of these recipes is to combine delicious flavors with digestive-friendly ingredients. Remembering these dinners for your eating regimen can give you a balanced way to support your stomach-related framework. It's fundamental to pay attention to your body and change recipes in view of individual inclinations and responsive qualities. Talking with a medical services professional or nutritionist can provide customized guidance in view of your particular dietary necessities and wellbeing objectives.

Meal Planning Tips for Promoting Stomach Wellness

Ways to advance stomach wellbeing include smart thought of the kinds of food sources, their readiness, and the general construction of your everyday meals. Through meal planning, consider the following practical hints to support stomach health.

Balanced Diet Principles: Incorporate an assortment of nutritional categories into every dinner, like organic products, vegetables, entire grains, lean proteins, and solid fats. Take a stab at an equilibrium of macronutrients (sugars, proteins, and fats) to give supported energy.

Fiber-Rich Foods: Consolidate high-fiber food varieties like entire grains, vegetables, organic products, and vegetables into your dinners. Slowly increase your fiber intake to allow your stomach-related framework to adjust.

Hydration: Hydrate over the course of the day to help with processing. Think about beginning your day with a glass of water to launch hydration.

Mindful Eating: Practice careful eating by focusing on appetite and completion signals. Bite food completely to support assimilation and supplement retention.

Probiotics and prebiotics: Incorporate probiotic-rich food sources like yogurt, kefir, sauerkraut, and kimchi to help build a solid stomach microbiome. Devour prebiotic food sources like bananas, garlic, and onions to sustain valuable stomach microbes.

Smaller, Frequent Meals: To avoid overtaxing the digestive system, choose smaller, more frequent meals throughout the day. This can help keep you from feeling bloated and uncomfortable after eating a lot of food.

Limit Processed Foods: Limit the admission of exceptionally handled and refined food sources, as they might contain added substances and additives that can be brutal on the stomach. Pick entire, natural food sources whenever the situation allows.

Limit Spicy and Fatty Foods: Lessen the utilization of hot and high-fat food varieties, as they might add to heartburn and indigestion. Pick milder flavors, and pick lean sources of fat.

Meal Timing: Space dinners equitably over the course of the day to keep up with steady energy levels. Keep away from weighty feasts near sleep time to forestall heartburn.

Individualized Approach: Identify and accommodate any particular food intolerances or sensitivities you may have. Try a variety of foods to find ones that are enjoyable and easy on the stomach.

Keep a Food Diary: Track your meals and note how your stomach feels subsequent to eating. Distinguish examples or trigger food sources that might be causing stomach-related distress.

Get professional advice: In the event that you have persistent stomach-related issues, talk with a medical services professional or an enlisted dietitian for customized direction and guidance.

Keep in mind that everybody's stomach-related framework is exceptional, and what works for one individual may not work for another. It is absolutely necessary to pay attention to the signals sent by your body, make adjustments based on your specific requirements, and seek professional guidance if necessary. The objective is to make a meal plan that upholds your general wellbeing and adds to an agreeable and well-working stomach-related framework.

Adapting Traditional Dishes to Enhance Stomach Function

Adapting Traditional Dishes to Enhance Stomach Function is adjusting meals to making smart alterations to recipes without forfeiting flavor or social importance. The objective is to make stomach-accommodating variants of cherished dishes that are delicate on the stomach-related framework. Traditional dishes can be altered in the following ways:

Introduction to Traditional Dishes:

Cultural Significance: Recognize the significance of customary dishes in different foods and the social associations they hold.

Balancing Act: Underline the need to offset social genuineness with stomach-related solace.

Healthy Modifications:

Ingredient Substitutions: Trade refined grains with entire grains (e.g., earthy-colored rice rather than white rice). Pick lean protein sources (e.g., chicken breast, turkey, and tofu) over greasy cuts of meat. Supplant saturated fats with better fats, like olive oil or avocado oil.

Reducing Added Sugars and Salt: Eliminate added sugars by utilizing normal sugars like honey or maple syrup. Use spices and flavors for flavor rather than over-the-top salt.

Incorporating More Vegetables: Increment the vegetable substance in dishes to support fiber and supplement admission. Try experimenting with a wide range of vibrant vegetables to improve nutrition and flavor.

Spice and Herb Alternatives:

Mild Spice Substitutes: Settle on milder flavors like cumin, coriander, or paprika rather than hot peppers. Utilize new spices like parsley, cilantro, or basil to add depth without overpowering the stomach.

Gentle Seasoning Techniques: Meal or barbecue as opposed to broiling to lessen the utilization of inordinate oils. Use citrus juices or vinegar-based marinades for a tasty, stomach-accommodating alternative.

Portion Control:

Moderation is Key: To avoid overeating and alleviate digestive stress, encourage mindful portion control. Give tips on paying attention to appetite and completion signs.

Customization for Specific Diets:

Gluten-Free or Dairy-Free Options: Offer choices for those with gluten or lactose awareness. Investigate without gluten-free flours, dairy choices, or plant-based choices.

Vegetarian or Vegan Variations:

Grandstand veggie lover or vegetarian variations of conventional meat-driven dishes. Feature plant-based proteins like beans, lentils, or tofu.

Cooking Techniques for Digestive Comfort:

Baking and steaming: To preserve nutrients without adding too much fat, encourage gentle cooking methods like baking and steaming. Share tips on keeping up with delicacies without compromising stomach health.

Broths and Soups: Consider soups and broths as stomach-friendly alternatives due to their hydrating properties and ease of digestion. Incorporate recipes for handcrafted stocks with stomach-related spices and flavors.

Family-Friendly Modifications:

Getting Kids Involved: Recommend family-accommodating variations to urge kids to appreciate stomach-accommodating dinners. Give imaginative plans for including kids in the cooking system.

Taste Testing and Feedback:

Encourage Experimentation: Welcome perusers to explore different avenues regarding adjusting their number one conventional recipe. Share a stage for perusers to give criticism and offer their fruitful transformations. Keep in mind to convey the idea that traditional dishes can be altered without compromising their essence. All things considered, it's tied in with settling on careful decisions to help stomach capability while still appreciating the rich social experience of adored feasts.

CHAPTER SIX

STOMACH CARE FOR DIFFERENT LIFE STAGES AND CONDITIONS

Stomach Care for Various Life Stages and Conditions includes fitting stomach-related wellbeing practices to meet the particular requirements and difficulties of people at different life stages or those encountering different medical issues. This will be checked under the following heading:

Special Considerations for Children, Seniors, and Pregnant Individuals

Special Considerations for Children, Seniors, and Pregnant Individuals as far as stomach-related wellbeing include perceiving the one-of-a kind requirements, difficulties, and potential dangers related to each group. For each demographic, specific considerations include:

1. Children:

a. Nutrient-Rich Diet: Significance of Development and Improvement: Underscore the requirement for an even, supplement-rich eating routine to help the fast development and advancement of children.

b. Hydration: Hydration Propensities: Support normal water consumption, particularly during proactive tasks and in a warm climate, to prevent dehydration.

c. Fiber Intake: Advancing Stomach-Related Consistency: Incorporate an assortment of fiber-rich food varieties like organic products, vegetables, and whole grains to help with stomach-related routineness.

d. Establishing Healthy Eating Habits: Role Modeling: In order to instill healthy eating habits that will last a lifetime, parents and other caregivers should be positive role models.

e. Food Allergy Awareness: recognizable proof, and the executives: Advance attention to normal food sensitivities and guide guardians in distinguishing and overseeing likely sensitivities or responsive qualities.

f. Avoiding Sugary and Processed Foods: Limiting Added Sugars: Promoter for restricted utilization of sweet and handled food varieties to forestall the early improvement of undesirable dietary propensities.

2. Seniors:

a. Hydration: Diminished Thirst Sensation: Address the likely reduction in thirst sensation in seniors by empowering standard water admission to forestall lack of hydration.

b. Dietary Fiber: Managing Constipation: Stress the significance of fiber in your diet for managing constipation, a common problem for older people.

c. Protein Admission: Keeping up with Bulk: Energize a satisfactory admission of protein to help muscle wellbeing and forestall age-related muscle misfortune.

d. Balancing Nutrient Needs: Nutrient and Mineral Admission: Advance an even eating regimen to guarantee seniors meet their supplement prerequisites, particularly for calcium, vitamin D, and B nutrients.

e. Medication and Digestive Health: Attention to Drugs Secondary effects: Bring issues to light about what medications might mean for stomach-related wellbeing and energize conversations with medical services suppliers.

f. Dental Health: Maintaining Oral Health: Take care of problems with your mouth because bad teeth can make it hard to chew and eat.

3. Pregnant Individuals:

a. Nutrient-Rich Diet: Expanded Supplement Needs: Stress the requirement for extra supplements during pregnancy, including folic acid, iron, calcium, and omega-3 unsaturated fats.

b. Hydration: Preventing Dehydration: To support increased blood volume and amniotic fluid, emphasize the significance of staying hydrated throughout pregnancy.

c. How to Handle Morning Sickness: Gentle Diet Modifications: For people who are experiencing morning sickness, suggest making dietary adjustments such as eating smaller, more frequent meals and bland, easy-to-digest foods.

d. Fiber Intake: Forestalling Clogging: Urge satisfactory fiber admission to forestall blockage, a typical issue during pregnancy.

e. Keeping Certain Foods Away: Sanitation Mindfulness: Give direction on keeping away from specific food varieties, for example, half-cooked meats and unpasteurized dairy, to decrease the risk of food borne ailments.

f. Managing Heartburn: Dietary Changes: Offer dietary methodologies to oversee indigestion, a typical worry during pregnancy, for example, by keeping away from huge dinners and acidic or hot food varieties.

g. Weight Management: Balanced Approach: Advocate for a well-balanced approach to weight gain during pregnancy, stressing the significance of meeting dietary requirements without overindulging in calories.

General Advice for Every Group:

Ordinary Check-ups: Advocate for ordinary check-ups with medical care experts to address particular wellbeing concerns and get customized counseling.

Individualized Approaches: Perceive that people inside these gatherings might have one-of-a kind dietary necessities and responsive qualities, and urge customized ways to deal with care.

Education and Communication: To address any digestive issues promptly, emphasize the significance of education and open communication with healthcare providers.

Lifestyle Factors:

Highlight the significance of way of life factors, for example, ordinary actual work, and stress the board for generally speaking stomach-related health across all life stages.

Extraordinary contemplations for children, seniors, and pregnant individuals include fitting dietary counsel and way of life proposals to accommodate the special requirements and difficulties related to each group. Individualized approaches, normal health check-ups, and open correspondence with medical services suppliers assume significant roles in advancing stomach-related health all through the different phases of life.

Stomach Care for Individuals with Chronic Health Conditions

Stomach care for people with ongoing medical issues includes a customized and designated way to deal with side effects, support, generally speaking, prosperity, and limit potential entanglements connected with their particular medical issue. The following are in-depth considerations for stomach care for people with chronic conditions:

1. Diabetes:

a. Blood Sugar Management:

Balanced Carbohydrate Intake: Empower a decent admission of carbohydrate, focusing on whole grains, natural products, and vegetables.

Regular Meal Timing: Elevate reliable dinner timing to assist with settling blood glucose levels over the course of the day.

a. Diet High in Fiber: Integrate fiber-rich food sources to help stomach-related wellbeing and direct glucose levels.

b. Segment Control: Moderation: Focus on portion control to help control blood sugar and prevent overeating.

c. Hydration: satisfactory Liquid Admission: Urge standard water admission to remain hydrated, as parchedness can influence glucose levels.

2. Inflammatory Bowel Disease (IBD - Crohn's Disease, Ulcerative Colitis):

a. Low-Fiber Diet During Flares: Low-Fiber Foods: During flares, a low-fiber diet is recommended to reduce digestive tract irritation. Supplement Supplementation: Consider supplementation to address expected supplement shortages because of malabsorption during flares.

b. Probiotics: Probiotic-rich food varieties or enhancements: Investigate the utilization of probiotics to assist with adjusting the stomach microbiome.

c. Prebiotics Food Sources: Incorporate prebiotics-rich food varieties to support helpful stomach microorganisms.

d. Hydration: Adequate Fluid Intake: Stress the significance of maintaining adequate hydration, particularly during flare-ups.

e. Individualized Triggers: ID of trigger food sources: Work with people to distinguish explicit trigger food varieties that might worsen side effects. Food Journal: Empower keeping a food journal to follow side effects and recognize designs.

3. Gastroesophageal Reflux Disease (GERD)::

a. Dietary Modifications: avoidance of foods that cause reflux It is suggested that acidic, spicy, and fatty foods be avoided. Little, Continuous Feasts: Energize more modest, more regular dinners to diminish tension on the lower esophageal sphincter.

b. Meal Timing: Keep away from Late-Evening Eating: Beat eating near sleep time to limit evening time reflux. Pose after dinners: Suggest remaining upstanding for a period after meals to lessen the risk of reflux.

c. Elevating Head During Sleep: Suggest hoisting the top of the bed to lessen evening side effects of lying head too low.

d. Weight Management: Keeping a Sound weight backing: endeavors to accomplish and keep a solid weight, as overabundance weight can add to reflux.

4. Gluten Intolerance:

a. Gluten-Free Diet: Severe Adherence to a Without Gluten Diet: Stress the significance of totally staying away from gluten-containing food varieties to oversee side effects. Schooling on Without Gluten Living: Give instruction on distinguishing without gluten choices and perusing food names.

b. Nutrient-Rich Substitutes: Picking Supplement Thick Other options: Assist people with finding supplement-rich choices for grains and food sources normally containing gluten.

c. Checking for Cross-Defilement: Understanding Marks: Urge careful name-perusing to distinguish possible wellsprings of gluten and limit the risk of cross-pollution.

d. Dietary Fiber Sources: Sans Gluten Fiber Sources: Give direction on non-gluten sources of dietary fiber to help stomach-related wellbeing.

Chronic Kidney Disease (CKD):

a. Controlling Protein Consumption:

Control of Protein Admission: Suggest a balance in protein consumption, especially in the high-level phases of CKD. Excellent Protein: Underline great protein sources to decrease the weight on the kidneys.

b. Phosphorus Control:

Phosphorus-Mindful Eating Routine: Backer for an eating routine that is aware of phosphorus content to oversee intricacies connected with CKD. Phosphorus

Binders: If necessary, collaborate with healthcare providers to manage phosphorus levels with medication.

c. Fluid Restriction: Checking Liquid Admission: For people with liquid limitations, screen and oversee liquid admission to forestall entanglements. **Hydration Management**: Team up with medical services suppliers to guarantee harmony among hydration and liquid limitations.

d. Individualized Nutrition Plans:: Cooperation with Dietitians: Energize coordinated effort with enlisted dietitians to make customized nourishment plans custom-made to explicit CKD stages.

General Tips for All Chronic Health Conditions:

Individualized Approaches: Be aware that each person may have particular dietary requirements and sensitivities associated with their particular chronic health condition.

Collaboration with Healthcare Providers: Support open correspondence with medical care suppliers, including dietitians, to guarantee an exhaustive and facilitated way to deal with care.

Regular Monitoring:

Ensure that symptoms and dietary habits are closely monitored on a regular basis to identify patterns and make any necessary adjustments.

Drug Contemplations:

Know about the likely effects of drugs on stomach-related wellbeing and team up with medical services suppliers to deal with any aftereffects.

Mindful Eating:

Advance careful eating rehearses, like biting food completely and focusing on appetite and totality signs.

Lifestyle Factors:

Feature the meaning of lifestyle factors like ordinary actual work and stress the board for in general stomach-related health.

A holistic and individualized approach to stomach care for people with chronic conditions includes dietary changes, lifestyle adjustments, and ongoing collaboration with healthcare professionals to improve digestive health and overall well-being.

Tailoring Stomach Care Approaches to Specific Needs

Ways to Deal with Explicit Requirements includes modifying methodologies and interventions to address the remarkable prerequisites, awareness, and difficulties of people in view of their particular medical issues, inclinations, and phases of life. This approach perceives that a one-size-fits-all way to deal with stomach care isn't reasonable, and customized contemplations are critical for compelling administration. Here is a comprehensive explanation of how to tailor stomach care to specific requirements:

1. Understanding Individual Health Conditions:

Evaluation and Conclusion: Start by understanding the individual's particular medical issue, whether it's an ongoing infection like diabetes, gastrointestinal problems, or other health concerns.

Medical History: Take into account the person's medical history, including any previous surgeries, medications, or gastrointestinal issues they may have.

2. Personalized Dietary Plans

Nutrient Requirements: Customize dietary plans to meet a person's unique nutrient needs based on their health status. For instance: Diabetes: underline adjusted starch admission and ordinary dinner timing. Celiac Sickness: Execute a severe gluten-free diet. Incendiary Inside Illness (IBD): Change fiber admission during eruptions.

3. Customizing Meal Timing and Frequency

Individual Schedules: When scheduling meal times and frequency, take into account each person's schedule and preferences. Persistent medical issue: People with conditions like GERD might profit from more modest, more successive dinners to forestall reflux.

4. Adapting to Cultural and Lifestyle Preferences

Social Contemplations: Regard and consolidate social dietary inclinations and limitations. Way of life elements: Address way of life factors, for example, work plans, actual work levels, and social commitment, while fitting stomach care draws near.

5. Managing Digestive Symptoms

Side effect acknowledgement: recognize explicit stomach-related side effects or issues that people might be aware of. Designated Mediations: Designers intercede to oversee and lighten these side effects. For instance, recommend dietary changes to reduce the causes of heartburn. Clogging: recommend fiber-rich food varieties and expanded liquid admission.

6. Taking Dietary Preferences into Account:

Vegetarian or Vegan Diets: change dietary intends to oblige vegan or vegetarian inclinations while guaranteeing satisfactory supplement admission. Food intolerances or allergies: Make adjustments to your diet to avoid certain foods.

7. Individualized Hydration Suggestions

Liquid Necessities: Consider individual liquid requirements in light of ailments, drugs, and action levels. Liquid Limitations: Adjust hydration proposals for people with liquid limitations because of conditions like constant kidney infections.

8. Medication Considerations

Influence on Stomach-Related Wellbeing: Know about drugs that might influence stomach-related wellbeing, like those causing blockage or heartburn. Time of Medication: If you want your medication to be as effective as possible and have as few side effects as possible, you should think about when you eat your meals.

9. Addressing Stress and Emotional Well-being

Mind-Body Association: Perceive the impact of weight on stomach-related wellbeing. Stress The board Methods: Designer proposals for stress decrease, which might incorporate care, unwinding activities, or guiding.

10. Promoting Consistent Follow-ups:

Standard Observing: Energize customary registrations and subsequent meet-ups to evaluate the viability of customized mediations. Changes, depending on the situation: Adjust stomach care approaches in view of progressing appraisals and criticism.

11. Educating and Empowering Individuals:

Healthful Instruction: Give customized, wholesome schooling, engaging people to settle on informed decisions. Taking care of oneself Procedures: Energize the improvement of taking care of oneself's systems and propensities that line up with individual necessities and inclinations.

12. Collaboration with Healthcare Professionals:

Multidisciplinary Approach: Place an emphasis on working together with healthcare professionals like primary care physicians, gastroenterologists, and dietitians. Medical, dietary, and lifestyle factors should all be taken into consideration when providing holistic stomach care.

13. Adapting as Needs Change:

Changes in Life Stages: Be aware that different life stages, such as pregnancy, aging, or changes in health status, may necessitate different needs for stomach care. Adaptable Plans: Plan adaptable plans that can be adjusted to advancing requirements and conditions.

14. Promoting Positive Eating Experiences:

Agreeable and Manageable: Designer stomach care ways to deal with make pleasant and feasible eating encounters. Culinary Preferences: To make stomach care a positive part of a person's overall well-being, think about their culinary preferences.

15. Encouraging a Holistic Approach:

Adjusting Elements: Elevate an all-encompassing way to deal with stomach care that tends to consider dietary perspectives as well as physical, profound, and social variables. Individual Objectives: Align stomach care methods with individual objectives for health and wellness. Fitting stomach care ways to deal with explicit necessities includes an extensive comprehension of a person's medical issue, inclinations, and way of life.

By modifying dietary plans, tending to side effects, considering social and way of life factors, and teaming up with medical services experts, custom-made stomach care turns into an essential piece of advancing, generally speaking, wellbeing and prosperity. This approach perceives the uniqueness of every person and endeavors to make practical and positive propensities that help stomach-related wellbeing all through different life stages and medical issues.

<h1 style="text-align:center">CHAPTER SEVEN</h1>

RECIPES FOR A HEALTHY DIGESTIVE SYSTEM

A. **Gut-Friendly Meals:** Stomach-agreeable dinners are feasts that are delicate on the stomach-related framework and provide sustenance. They usually focus on foods that are easier to digest and less likely to cause IBS symptoms. The following are some key components of gut-friendly meals:

Lean proteins: Choose proteins like chicken, fish, tofu, or lentils that are low in fat. These are more straightforward to process compared with higher-fat choices. Cooked vegetables: Cooking vegetables can assist with separating their strands, making them more straightforward to process. Steamed or cooked vegetables like carrots, zucchini, or chile peppers are extraordinary decisions.

Whole grains: Pick entire grains like earthy-colored rice, quinoa, or oats that are high in fiber but gentler on the stomach-related framework. Stay away from refined grains, as they might have side effects.

Healthy fats: Incorporate limited quantities of solid fats like avocado, olive oil, or nuts. These can add flavor and satiety to your dinners without overburdening the stomach-related framework.

Low FODMAP options: If you eat a low-FODMAP diet, you should choose foods that don't have many fermentable carbohydrates (FODMAPs). This can assist with diminishing gas, bulging, and other IBS side effects.

B. Smoothies and Digestive Elixirs: Smoothies and digestive elixirs can support digestion and supply essential nutrients in a convenient manner.

When making these drinks, consider the following:

Ingredients high in fiber: To increase fiber intake, include ingredients like spinach, kale, chia seeds, or flaxseeds. Nonetheless, be careful in the event that you're sensitive to high-fiber food varieties.

Hydrating base: Pick a hydrating base like water, coconut water, or a low-sugar almond milk. These can assist with keeping up with hydration and supporting assimilation.

Probiotic sources: Add wellsprings of probiotics like Greek yogurt or kefir to advance a solid stomach microbiome. Choose alternatives that do not contain dairy if you are lactose intolerant or have a dairy allergy.

Digestive-friendly herbs and spices: Examination with spices and flavors like ginger, mint, fennel, or turmeric. These can soothe the stomach-related framework and add flavor to your elixirs.

Personalize to your needs: Designer your smoothies or elixirs as you would prefer inclinations and dietary limitations. Go ahead and investigate various blends and fixings, remembering what turns out best for your body.

C. **Snack Ideas for Better Digestion**: Eating can be an incredible chance to help with assimilation and provide support for energy over the course of the day. Snacks that are gentle on the digestive system include the following:

Rice cakes or gluten-free crackers with almond butter or hummus spread are both low in fat and easy to digest, making them a healthy snack option. Yogurt with low-FODMAP natural products: Settle on plain yogurt (Greek or sans dairy choices) and add low-FODMAP natural products like strawberries, blueberries, or kiwi for additional flavor and fiber.

Boiled Eggs: Eggs are a decent source of protein and can be a fantastic tidbit. They are also generally well-tolerated by most people.

Baked sweet potato fries: Slice sweet potatoes into fries, lightly coat them with olive oil, and bake until crispy. Sweet potatoes are nutritious and more straightforward to process than ordinary potatoes.

Smoothie bowls: Make a smoothie bowl with a mix of low-FODMAP natural products, a protein source like almond spread or pea protein powder, and a little modest bunch of sans-gluten granola or nuts for added surface.

Rice pudding: Cook rice in sans lactose milk or a dairy-free alternative, add a hint of maple syrup, and sprinkle with cinnamon. This smooth and somewhat sweet treat can be delicate on the stomach.

Homemade trail mix: Make a blend of low-FODMAP nuts like almonds or pecans, alongside seeds like pumpkin or sunflower seeds, and a modest quantity of low-FODMAP dried natural products like cranberries or coconut pieces.

Keep in mind that these are just some ideas; you can modify them to meet your particular dietary requirements. It's generally really smart to talk with a medical services proficient or enrolled dietitian for customized counsel in light of your unique circumstances.

CHAPTER EIGHT

SUPPLEMENTS AND DIGESTIVE HEALTH

A. **Traditional Medicine Practices**: Conventional medication practices, like Ayurveda and customary Chinese medicine (TCM), have long perceived the significance of stomach-related wellbeing. These practices adopt an all-encompassing strategy by thinking about the body, brain, and soul as interconnected. Customary medication frequently utilizes spices, dietary suggestions, and explicit strategies to advance stomach-related health.

In Ayurveda, the attention is on adjusting the three doshas (Vata, Pitta, and Kapha) to keep up with ideal processing. Ayurvedic spices like ginger, turmeric, and fennel are ordinarily used to aid assimilation. Dietary suggestions, like eating warm, cooked food sources and staying away from in-congruent food blends, are additionally underscored.

TCM sees absorption as an interaction that includes the change and transportation of supplements. Irregular characteristics in the body's energy, known as Qi, can prompt stomach-related issues. TCM utilizes different spices, needle therapy, and dietary alterations to reestablish harmony and advance solid absorption. Ginger, licorice, and dandelion root, for instance, can be used to treat specific digestive issues.

B. **Mind-Body Connection**: The brain-body association features the impact of our viewpoints, feelings, and feelings of anxiety on our actual prosperity, including stomach-related wellbeing. Stress, uneasiness, and other gloomy feelings can influence the stomach-related framework, prompting side effects like acid reflux, swelling, and modified solid discharges.

Rehearses like care, reflection, and profound breathing activities can assist with decreasing feelings of anxiety and advance unwinding, consequently emphatically influencing assimilation. These procedures urge us to be available, tune into our bodies, and develop a feeling of quiet. By overseeing pressure and cultivating a positive outlook, we can uphold better processing.

C. **Integrative Methodologies**: Integrative ways to deal with stomach-related health include consolidating regular medication with reciprocal treatments to address the entire individual. This approach perceives that actual wellbeing is impacted by natural elements as well as by way of life, close-to-home prosperity, and ecological variables. Integrative methodologies might include working with a medical care group that incorporates clinical specialists, enrolled dietitians, naturopathic specialists, and different experts. They might use a blend of medicines, like dietary changes, supplements, natural cures, stress management methods, and brain-body exercises, to work on stomach-related wellbeing.

By adopting an integrative strategy, people can profit from the smartest possible situation by joining proof-based regular medication with corresponding practices that address the underlying drivers of stomach-related issues. The goal of this strategy is to improve digestion and overall health.

Keep in mind that it's dependably essential to talk with a medical services expert prior to attempting any new ways to help your stomach-related wellbeing. They can give customized counsel in view of your particular necessities and clinical history.

Moreover, keeping a solid way of life can essentially affect your stomach-related prosperity. A few general ways to advance great processing include:

Maintaining a well-balanced diet means eating a variety of fruits and vegetables, whole grains, lean proteins, and healthy fats. Eat foods high in fiber to encourage regular bowel movements.

Drinking a lot of water: Remaining hydrated helps in keeping up with solid processing and forestalling clogging.

Managing stress: Participate in exercises that assist you with unwinding, like yoga, reflection, or investing energy in nature. Track down solid ways of adapting to pressure to stay away from superfluous burdens on your stomach-related framework.

Regular exercise: Moving your body helps your digestion and improves your overall health. Hold back nothing—30 minutes of moderate-power practice most days of the week.

Keeping away from extreme liquor and smoking: These propensities can adversely affect assimilation and general wellbeing. Limit liquor utilization and, if conceivable, quit smoking.

Keep in mind that everybody's stomach-related framework is extraordinary, and what works for one individual may not work for another. It's fundamental to pay attention to your body, focus on any side effects or examples, and make changes appropriately.

Individuals are given the ability to address digestive issues holistically through integrative approaches, which incorporate both conventional and alternative treatments. Dietary treatment, including customized nourishment plans and eating less, offers designated help for stomach-related conditions. The way to progress lies in an individualized and cooperative methodology, coordinating these all-encompassing practices into one's way of life while working intimately with medical services experts.

CHAPTER NINE

CASE STUDIES AND SUCCESS STORIES

A. Personal Experiences with Digestive Health:

Case Study A: Sarah's Journey with Irritable Bowel Syndrome (IBS)

Sarah struggled with symptoms like abdominal pain, bloating, and irregular bowel movements for years. She sought medical help and was diagnosed with IBS.

Through a process of elimination, she identified trigger foods and made dietary adjustments. Sarah found relief by incorporating stress-reduction techniques like yoga and meditation into her daily routine.

Case Study B: Mark's Battle with Acid Reflux

Mark experienced frequent heartburn and regurgitation, affecting his quality of life.

After consulting with a gastroenterologist, he made lifestyle changes like avoiding spicy and fatty foods, quitting smoking, and elevating the head of his bed.

With the combination of medication and these adjustments, Mark's acid reflux symptoms significantly improved, allowing him to enjoy meals and sleep comfortably.

B. Success Stories

Success Stories 1: Emily's Triumph Over Crohn's Disease

Emily was diagnosed with Crohn's disease, experiencing severe abdominal pain, diarrhea, and fatigue.

She decided to follow a specific anti-inflammatory diet recommended by her doctor. Alongside dietary changes, she incorporated regular exercise and stress management techniques into her routine.

Over time, Emily's symptoms reduced, and she achieved remission, allowing her to live a fulfilling life.

Success Stories 2: Alex's Success with Food Intolerances

Alex struggled with ongoing digestive issues and suspected food intolerances.

He worked closely with a registered dietitian to identify trigger foods and develop a personalized elimination diet.

By eliminating certain foods and slowly reintroducing them, Alex discovered the specific culprits causing his symptoms.

Armed with this knowledge, he now enjoy a varied diet while avoiding trigger foods, improving his overall digestive health.

These practical examples provide a glimpse into the diverse experiences individuals have had with digestive health challenges and how they found effective solutions.

Remember, everyone's journey is unique, and it's essential to consult with healthcare professionals for personalized advice and guidance.

CHAPTER TEN

CONCLUSION

A. Recap of Stomach Solution Principles

All through our discussion about stomach-related health, we investigated different individual encounters and examples of overcoming adversity. Now, let's recap the key principles that emerged from these discussions:

Appropriate Dietary Administration: Numerous stomach-related conditions can be managed by focusing on what we eat. Recognizing trigger food sources, following explicit weight control plans suggested by medical care experts, and making dietary changes are fundamental stages towards tracking down alleviation.

Way of life Adjustments: Beyond diet, making lifestyle changes can have a significant impact on our digestive health. Methodologies like pressure decrease procedures, standard activity, and staying away from hurtful propensities (like smoking or extreme liquor utilization) can add to working on and large stomach-related prosperity.

Seeking Medical Advice: It's vital to talk with medical services experts, like gastroenterologists or enrolled dietitians, for a precise finding and customized direction.

They have the ability to assist with distinguishing hidden causes, suggest suitable medicines, and provide support all through your excursion.

B. Encouragement for a Healthy Digestive Lifestyle

Maintaining a healthy digestive lifestyle is essential for overall well-being. Here are some uplifting statements to move you en route:

Embrace a fair eating routine: By integrating various organic products—vegetables, entire grains, lean proteins, and solid fats—into your dinners, you can give your stomach-related framework vital supplements. Keep in mind that control is vital! Slow down, chew your food thoroughly, and savor each bite.

Practice Mindful Eating: This careful way to deal with eating can upgrade absorption and assist you with perceiving your body's signs of craving and completion.

Focus on the stomach. Well-disposed food sources: Probiotic-rich food sources like yogurt, kefir, sauerkraut, and kimchi can advance a sound stomach microbiome.

Also, fiber-rich food varieties like vegetables, entire grains, and organic products assist with supporting customary solid discharges.

Remain Hydrated: Drinking a satisfactory amount of water keeps up with ideal assimilation and prevents stoppage. Hold back nothing—eight cups of water each day; however, change in view of individual necessities.

Manage Stress: Constant pressure can adversely affect absorption. Track down and decrease procedures that work for you, for example, care activities, yoga, or participating in leisure activities that give you pleasure and unwind.

Listen to Your Body: Focus on any progressions or constant side effects, and talk with medical care experts if necessary. Trust your instinct and make strides towards advancing your stomach-related wellbeing. Keep in mind that it's an excursion, and little changes can have a major effect. Celebrate your progress.

www.ingramcontent.com/pod-product-compliance
Lightning Source LLC
Chambersburg PA
CBHW070750250726

48662CB00004B/1719